POCKET ATLAS OF
CARDIAC AND THORACIC MRI

D1705276

Pocket Atlas of Cardiac and Thoracic MRI

Jeffrey J. Brown, M.D.
Assistant Professor of Radiology
The Edward Mallinckrodt Institute of Radiology
St. Louis, Missouri

Charles B. Higgins, M.D.
Professor of Radiology
Chief, Magnetic Resonance Imaging
University of California
San Francisco, California

Raven Press New York

Raven Press, 1185 Avenue of the Americas, New York, New York 10036

Made in the United States of America

Library of Congress Cataloging-in-Publication Data

Brown, Jeffrey J.
  Pocket atlas of cardiac and thoracic MRI.

  Includes bibliographies and index.
  1. Heart—Magnetic resonance imaging—Atlases. 2. Chest—Magnetic resonance imaging—Atlases. 3. Heart—Magnetic resonance imaging—Handbooks, manuals, etc. 4. Chest—Magnetic resonance imaging—Handbooks, manuals, etc. I. Higgins, Charles B. [DNLM: 1. Heart—anatomy & histology—atlases. 2. Heart—pathology—atlases. 3. Heart Diseases—diagnosis—atlases. 4. Magnetic Resonance Imaging—atlases. 5. Thoracic Diseases—diagnosis—atlases. 6. Thorax—anatomy & histology—atlases. 7. Thorax—pathology—atlases. WG 17 B8783p]
RC670.5.M33B76   1989   616.1′20757   88-42584
ISBN 0-88167-488-5

The material contained in this volume was submitted as previously unpublished material, except in the instances in which credit has been given to the source from which some of the illustrative material was derived.

Great care has been taken to maintain the accuracy of the information contained in the volume. However, neither Raven Press nor the editors can be held responsible for errors or for any consequences arising from the use of the information contained herein.

9 8 7 6 5 4 3 2 1

Preface

MR imaging, with its ability to provide a detailed, composite view of chest anatomy in a noninvasive manner, has become a powerful new tool in the evaluation of cardiac and thoracic disease. Advantages of MR imaging include a lack of ionizing radiation, the ability to directly acquire images in multiple planes, and clear delineation of the cardiac chambers and great vessels without the need for intravenous contrast material.

With recent advances in MR technology, high quality thoracic and cardiac images are now being obtained at a variety of different magnetic field strengths. Anatomic images acquired at medium and high field strength are included in this pocket atlas. The medium field strength images were obtained with a 0.35 Tesla Diasonics MT/S imaging system. The high field strength images were acquired using a 1.5 Tesla General Electric Signa system. Gradient echo images were obtained on the Signa unit using gradient refocussed acquisition in the steady state (GRASS). These images are analogous to gradient echo images produced by other manufacturers under different acronyms (e.g., FLASH, FISP).

In addition to the standard orthogonal views (i.e., transaxial, coronal, and sagittal planes), the anatomy is displayed in planes related to the cardiac axis. The long axis of the left ventricle transects the middle of the aortic valve and the left ventricular apex. Short axis and long axis views of the heart, which are acquired perpendicular and parallel to the long axis of the left ventricle respectively, are demonstrated.

The concluding section is comprised of MR images of a variety of cardiac and thoracic abnormalities. This section illustrates the capability of MR imaging to clearly delineate pathologic conditions in the thorax.

The global depiction of anatomy in different planes afforded by MR imaging results in a large amount of anatomic information on each cardiac or thoracic MR examination. The purpose of this pocket atlas is to display this anatomy in a clear and concise manner to facilitate the interpretation of MR images and provide a practical and manageable guide to the anatomy of this region.

Contents

Normal
Anatomy _____

Medium Field Strength (0.35 T)
1, right brachiocephalic vein
2, medial head of clavicle
3, trachea
4, brachiocephalic artery
5, left common carotid artery
6, left brachiocephalic vein
7, left subclavian artery
8, esophagus
9, subscapularis muscle
10, infraspinatus muscle
11, third thoracic vertebra

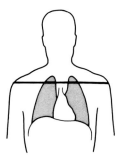

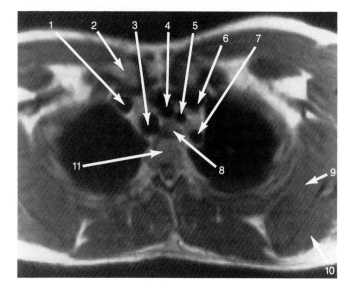

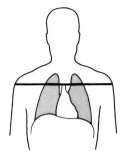

Medium Field Strength (0.35 T)
1, right brachiocephalic vein
2, left brachiocephalic vein
3, aortic arch
4, trapezius muscle
5, rhomboideus major muscle
6, spinal cord
7, trachea

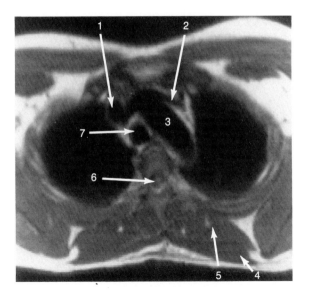

Medium Field Strength (0.35 T)
1, internal mammary vessels
2, aortic arch
3, rhomboideus major muscle
4, dorsal semispinalis and multifidus
   muscles
5, trachea
6, superior vena cava

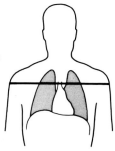

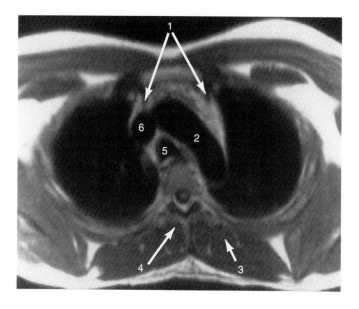

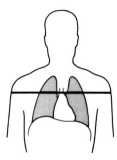

Medium Field Strength (0.35 T)
1, ascending aorta
2, pectoralis major muscle
3, pectoralis minor muscle
4, trachea
5, esophagus
6, descending aorta
7, azygos vein
8, superior vena cava

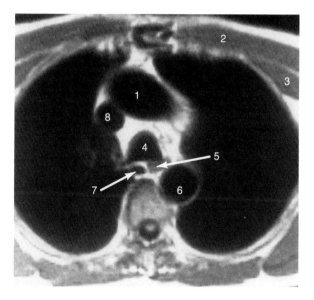

Medium Field Strength (0.35 T)
1, ascending aorta
2, main pulmonary artery
3, carina
4, descending aorta
5, right upper lobe bronchus
6, truncus anterior
7, superior vena cava

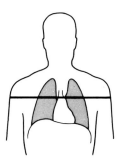

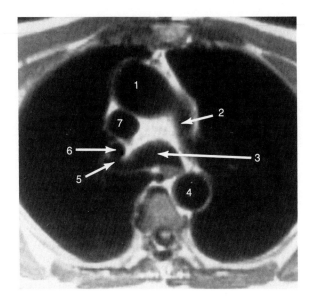

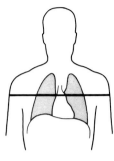

Medium Field Strength (0.35 T)
1, ascending aorta
2, main pulmonary artery
3, left pulmonary artery
4, descending aorta
5, longissimus dorsi muscle
6, dorsal semispinalis and
   multifidus muscles
7, trapezeus muscle
8, right main bronchus
9, right pulmonary artery
10, superior vena cava

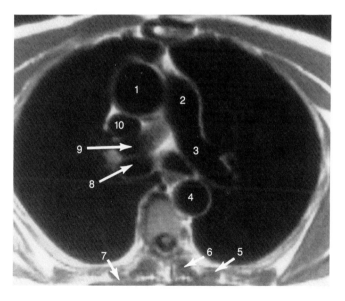

Medium Field Strength (0.35 T)
1, ascending aorta
2, main pulmonary artery
3, left atrial appendage
4, left superior pulmonary vein
5, left upper lobe bronchus
6, descending aorta
7, serratus anterior muscle
8, teres major muscle
9, latissimus dorsi muscle
10, azygos vein
11, bronchus intermedius
12, right pulmonary artery
13, superior vena cava

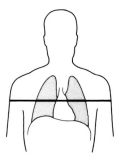

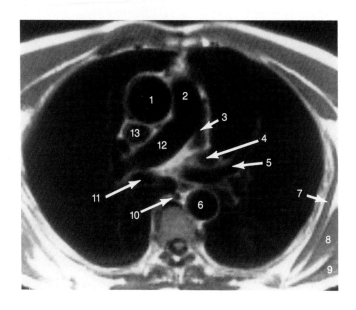

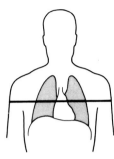

Medium Field Strength (0.35 T)
1, main pulmonary artery
2, left atrial appendage
3, left superior pulmonary vein
4, descending aorta
5, left atrium
6, right superior pulmonary vein
7, superior vena cava
8, ascending aorta

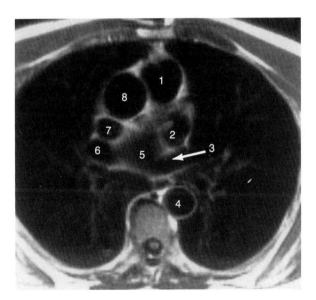

Medium Field Strength (0.35 T)
1, right ventricular outflow region
2, left coronary artery
3, pectoralis major muscle
4, left atrium
5, descending aorta
6, serratus anterior muscle
7, latissimus dorsi muscle
8, azygos vein
9, superior vena cava
10, ascending aorta

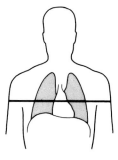

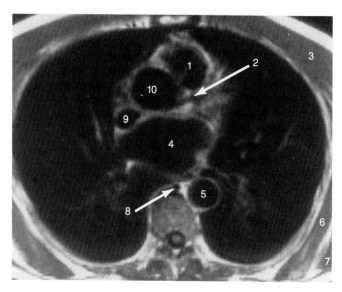

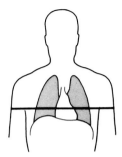

Medium Field Strength (0.35 T)
1, right ventricular outflow region
2, level of aortic valve
3, left atrium
4, left inferior pulmonary vein
5, descending aorta
6, right inferior pulmonary vein
7, junction of superior vena cava and right atrium
8, right atrial appendage
9, right coronary artery

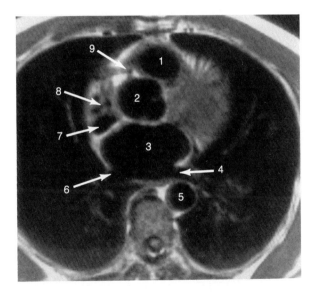

Medium Field Strength (0.35 T)
1, right ventricle
2, left ventricular outflow region
3, left ventricle
4, left atrium
5, descending aorta
6, right atrium

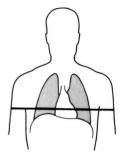

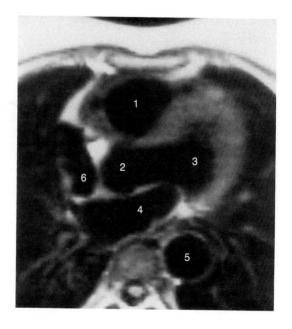

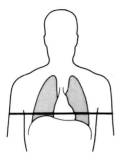

Medium Field Strength (0.35 T)
1, right ventricle
2, left ventricle
3, descending aorta
4, thoracic vertebra
5, spinal cord
6, azygos vein
7, left atrium
8, right atrium

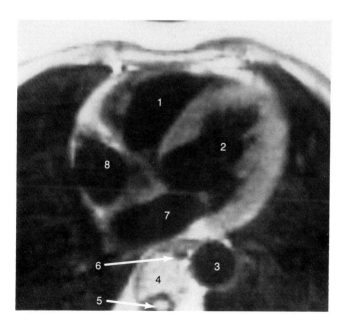

Medium Field Strength (0.35 T)
1, right ventricle
2, left ventricle
3, descending aorta
4, spinal cord
5, azygos vein
6, right atrium
7, tricuspid valve
8, right coronary artery
9, pericardium

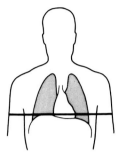

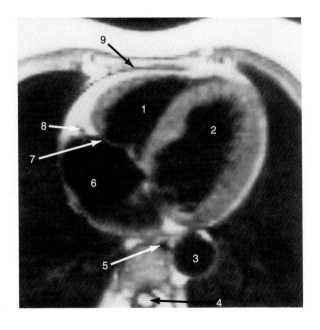

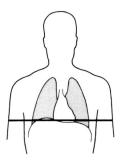

Medium Field Strength (0.35 T)
1, pericardium
2, right ventricle
3, left ventricle
4, papillary muscle
5, descending aorta
6, coronary sinus
7, right atrium

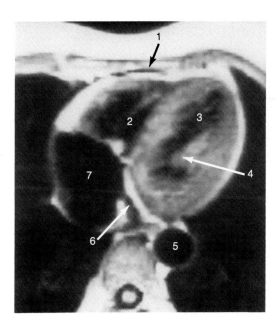

Medium Field Strength (0.35 T)
1, right ventricle
2, left ventricle
3, descending aorta
4, hemiazygos vein
5, azygos vein
6, esophagus
7, inferior vena cava

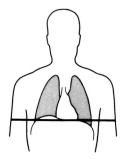

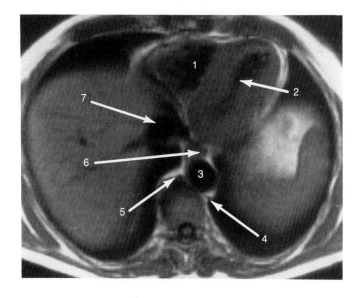

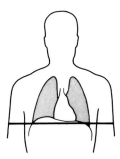

Medium Field Strength (0.35 T)
1, cardiac apex
2, distal esophagus
3, descending aorta
4, spleen
5, inferior vena cava
6, right hepatic vein
7, middle hepatic vein

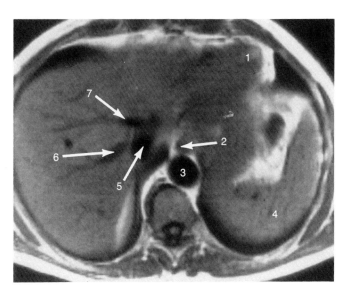

**Medium Field Strength (0.35 T)—
5-mm slice**
1, right ventricle
2, left descending pulmonary artery
3, descending aorta
4, left atrium
5, aortic valve cusps
6, right atrial appendage

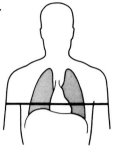

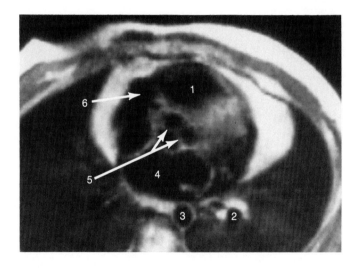

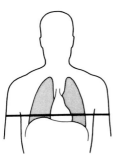

**Medium Field Strength
(0.35 T)—5-mm slice**
1, right ventricle
2, left ventricle
3, papillary muscle
4, pericardium
5, mitral valve
6, descending aorta
7, left atrium
8, right atrium

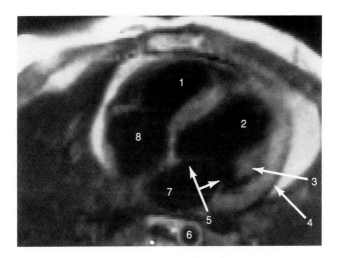

**Medium Field Strength (0.35 T)—
Normal Thymus in a
5-Year-Old Boy**

1, thymus
2, ascending aorta
3, main pulmonary artery
4, left pulmonary artery
5, left main bronchus
6, descending aorta
7, azygos vein
8, right main bronchus
9, right pulmonary artery
10, superior vena cava

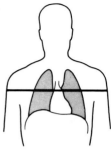

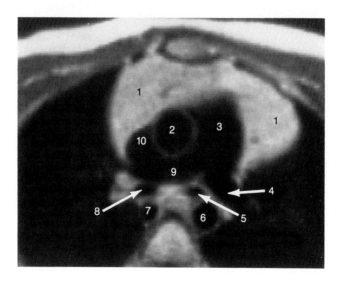

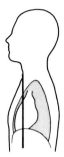

Medium Field Strength (0.35 T)
1, right ventricular outflow region
2, left ventricle
3, right ventricle

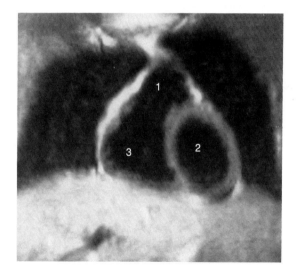

Medium Field Strength (0.35 T)
1, trachea
2, left brachiocephalic vein
3, aortic arch
4, main pulmonary artery
5, left atrial appendage
6, left ventricle
7, aorta
8, right atrium
9, right atrial appendage
10, right brachiocephalic vein
11, right subclavian vein
12, right internal jugular vein
13, right common carotid artery
14, brachiocephalic artery

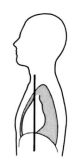

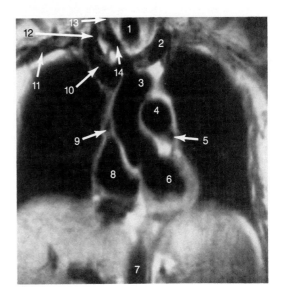

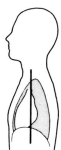

Medium Field Strength (0.35 T)
1, right subclavian artery
2, brachiocephalic artery
3, trachea
4, left common carotid artery
5, left subclavian artery
6, aortic arch
7, main pulmonary artery
8, great cardiac vein
9, left atrium
10, coronary sinus
11, aorta
12, inferior vena cava
13, right atrium
14, superior vena cava

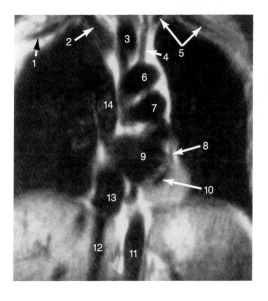

Medium Field Strength (0.35 T)

1, trachea
2, left subclavian artery
3, aortic arch
4, left pulmonary artery
5, left atrium
6, aorta
7, azygos vein
8, right pulmonary artery
9, arch of azygos vein

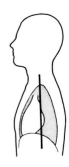

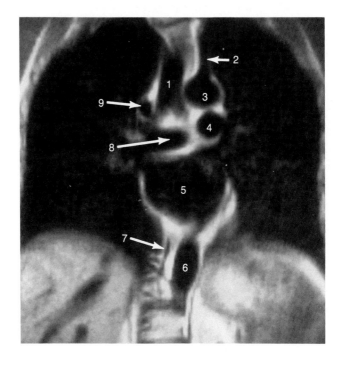

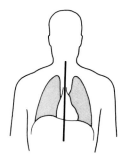

Medium Field Strength (0.35 T)
1, left brachiocephalic vein
2, trachea
3, ascending aorta
4, right pulmonary artery
5, left atrium
6, left ventricle
7, descending aorta
8, right ventricle
9, lung (right upper lobe)

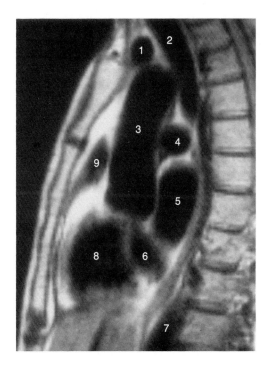

Medium Field Strength (0.35 T)
1, left brachiocephalic vein
2, left common carotid artery
3, aortic arch
4, origin of left main bronchus
5, right pulmonary artery
6, left atrium
7, descending aorta
8, right ventricle
9, left ventricular outflow region

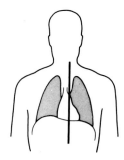

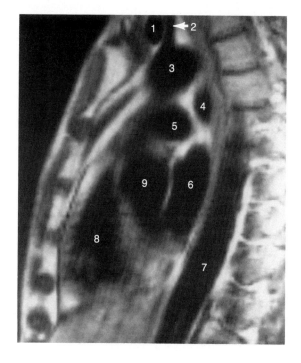

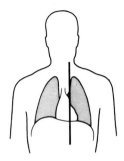

Medium Field Strength (0.35 T)
1, left brachiocephalic vein
2, left subclavian artery
3, aortic arch
4, left main bronchus
5, left atrium
6, left ventricle
7, right ventricle
8, lung (left upper lobe)
9, main pulmonary artery

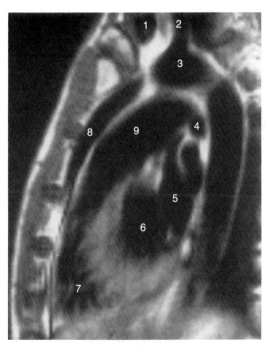

**Spin Echo Image in
the Sagittal Oblique
(LAO Equivalent)
Projection/Medium Field
Strength (0.35 T)**

1, aortic arch
2, main pulmonary artery
3, left pulmonary artery
4, left superior pulmonary vein
5, left main bronchus
6, left atrium
7, left ventricle
8, right ventricle
9, left brachiocephalic vein

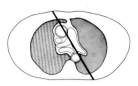

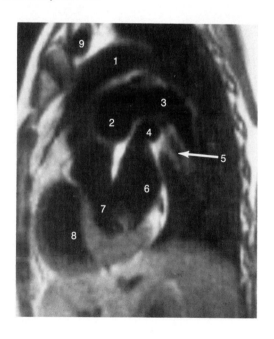

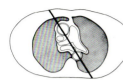

Spin Echo Image in the Sagittal Oblique (LAO Equivalent) Projection/ Medium Field Strength (0.35 T)

1, left common carotid artery
2, left subclavian artery
3, aortic arch
4, left main bronchus
5, left superior pulmonary vein
6, left inferior pulmonary vein
7, left atrium
8, coronary sinus
9, right ventricle
10, right atrial appendage
11, lung (right upper lobe)
12, left brachiocephalic vein

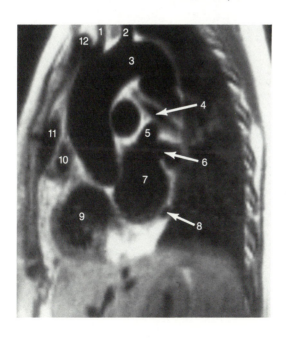

Spin Echo Image in the Sagittal Oblique (LAO Equivalent) Projection/ Medium Field Strength (0.35 T)

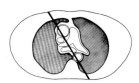

1, trachea
2, aorta
3, left main bronchus
4, right pulmonary artery
5, left atrium
6, atrial septum
7, right atrium
8, lung

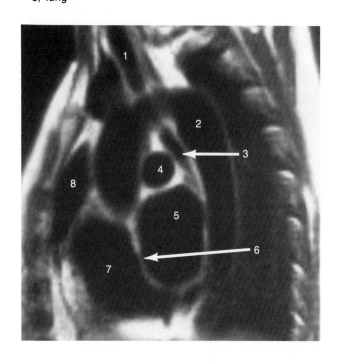

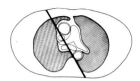

Spin Echo Image in the Sagittal Oblique (LAO Equivalent) Projection/ Medium Field Strength (0.35 T)

1, left brachiocephalic vein
2, trachea
3, right pulmonary artery
4, left atrium
5, aorta
6, right atrium
7, lung
8, superior vena cava
9, right inferior thyroid vein

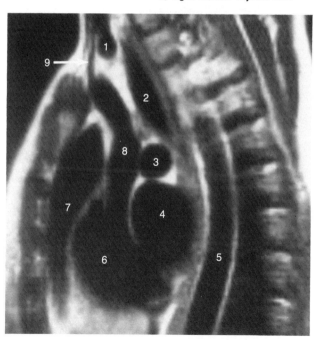

High Field Strength (1.5 T)
1, internal mammary artery and vein
2, ascending aorta
3, main pulmonary artery
4, left superior pulmonary vein
5, left main bronchus
6, descending aorta
7, right main bronchus
8, right superior pulmonary vein
9, superior vena cava

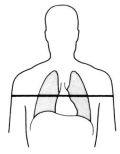

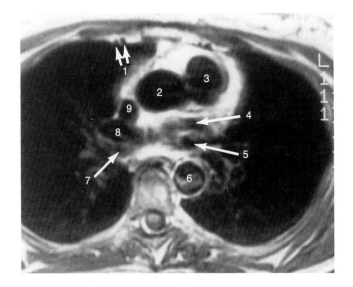

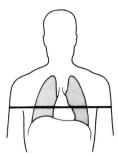

High Field Strength (1.5 T)
1, right ventricle
2, level of aortic valve
3, left ventricle
4, left circumflex coronary artery
5, left inferior pulmonary vein
6, descending aorta
7, left atrium
8, right atrium

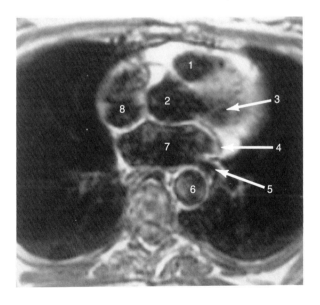

High Field Strength (1.5 T)
1, right ventricle
2, left ventricle
3, papillary muscle
4, descending aorta
5, azygos vein
6, right inferior pulmonary vein
7, left atrium
8, right atrium

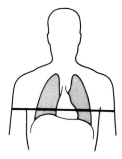

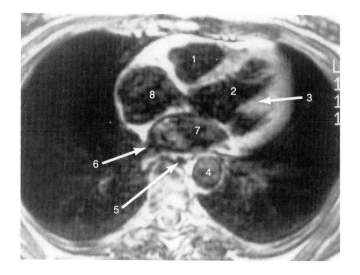

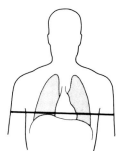

High Field Strength (1.5 T)
1, right ventricle
2, left ventricle
3, descending aorta
4, left atrium
5, right atrium
6, right coronary artery

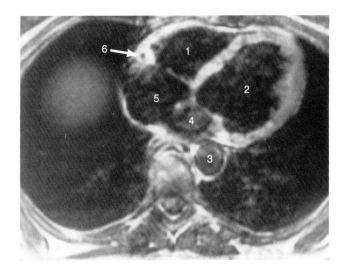

High Field Strength (1.5 T)
1, right ventricle
2, left ventricle
3, pericardium
4, descending aorta
5, azygos vein
6, coronary sinus
7, right atrium
8, dome of liver

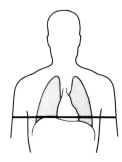

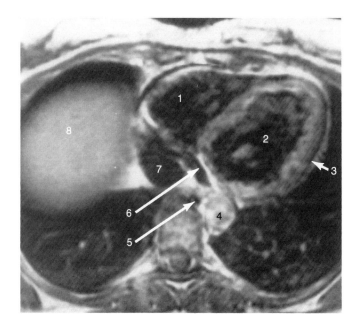

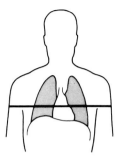

High Field Strength (1.5 T)
1, right ventricle
2, aortic valve
3, left atrium
4, descending aorta
5, azygos vein
6, junction of superior vena cava
   and right atrium
7, right atrial appendage

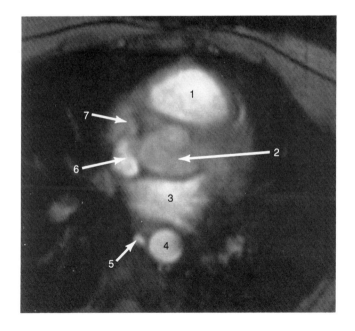

High Field Strength (1.5 T)
1, right ventricle
2, left ventricular outflow region
3, left atrium
4, left inferior pulmonary vein
5, descending aorta
6, azygos vein
7, right atrium

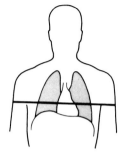

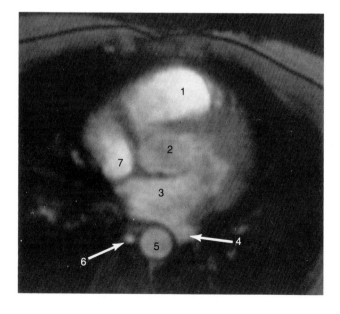

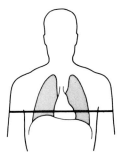

High Field Strength (1.5 T)
1, right ventricle
2, left ventricle
3, mitral valve
4, descending aorta
5, left atrium
6, right atrium
7, tricuspid valve

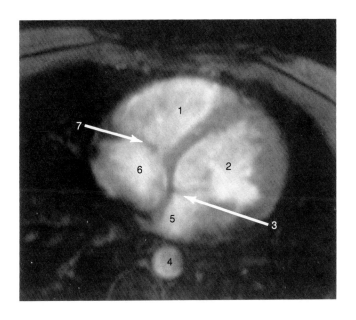

High Field Strength (1.5 T)

1, internal mammary artery and vein
2, right ventricle
3, moderator band of right ventricle
4, left ventricle
5, descending aorta
6, right atrium

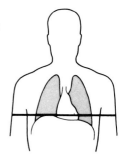

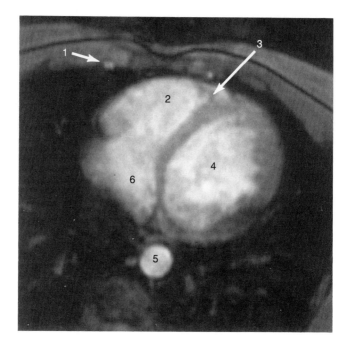

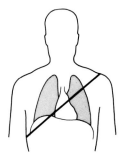

High Field Strength (1.5 T)— Short-Axis View
1, main pulmonary artery
2, ascending aorta
3, left atrium
4, descending aorta
5, right atrium

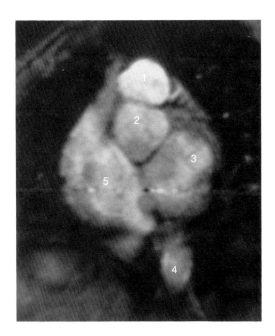

42

GRASS Image

**High Field Strength (1.5 T)—
Short-Axis View (Diastole)**
1, right ventricle
2, ventricular septum
3, left anterior descending coronary
   artery
4, left ventricle
5, papillary muscle
6, descending aorta
7, inferior vena cava

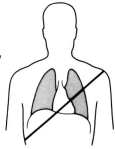

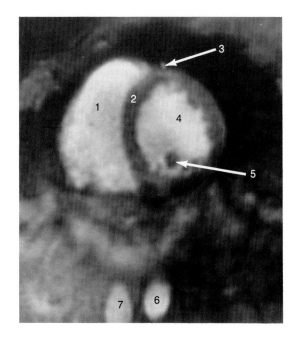

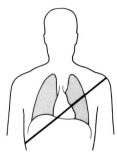

**High Field Strength (1.5 T)—
Short-Axis View (Systole)**
1, right ventricle
2, left anterior descending
   coronary artery
3, left ventricle
4, descending aorta
5, inferior vena cava

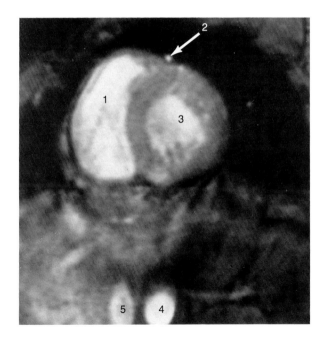

High Field Strength (1.5 T)— Long-Axis View
1, right ventricle
2, left ventricle
3, left atrium
4, descending aorta

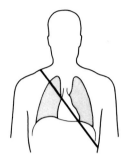

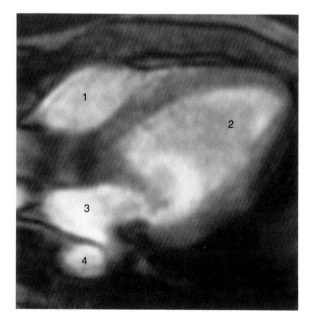

Abnormal Cases

**Medium Field Strength (0.35 T)—
Transaxial View**
1, aortic arch
2, persistent left superior vena cava
3, trachea

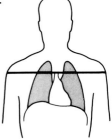

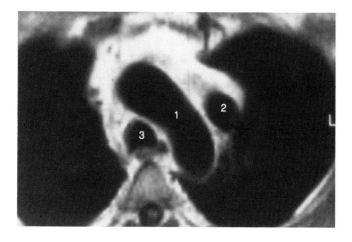

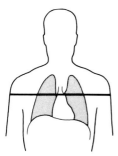

**Medium Field Strength
(0.35 T)—Transaxial View**
1, ascending aorta
2, main pulmonary artery
3, persistent left superior
vena cava
5, descending aorta
6, right main bronchus
7, truncus anterior
8, superior pericardial sinus

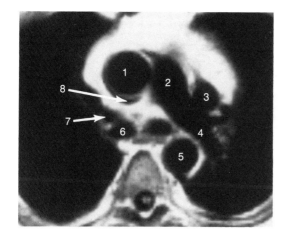

**Medium Field Strength (0.35 T)—
Transaxial View**
1, right ventricle
2, left ventricle
3, dilated vertical limb of coronary
   sinus
4, left atrium

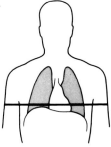

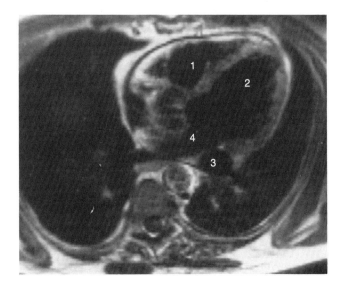

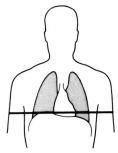

**Medium Field Strength
(0.35 T)—Transaxial View**
1, right ventricle
2, left ventricle
3, dilated coronary sinus
4, hemiazygos vein
5, dome of liver
6, right atrium

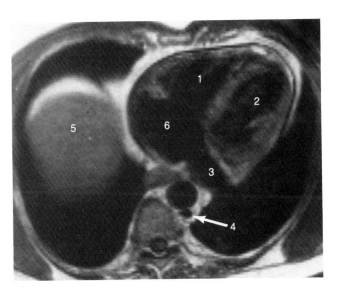

**Medium Field Strength (0.35 T)—
Coronal View**
1, trachea
2, aortic arch
3, persistent left superior vena cava
4, left pulmonary artery
5, left atrium
6, coronary sinus
7, right atrium
8, right superior pulmonary vein
9, right pulmonary artery

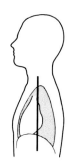

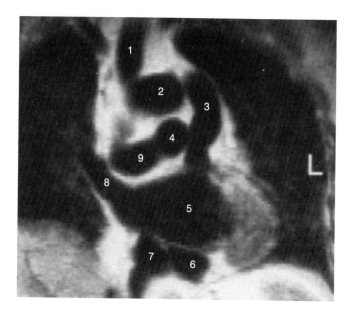

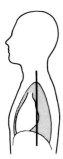

**Medium Field Strength (0.35 T)—
Coronal View**
1, aortic arch
2, left pulmonary artery
3, left superior pulmonary vein
4, left atrium
5, dilated coronary sinus
6, right inferior pulmonary vein
7, right main bronchus

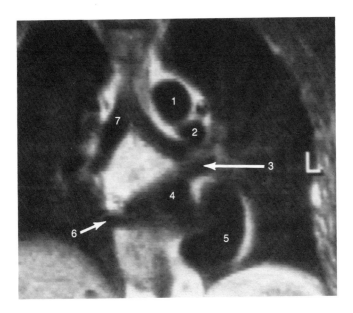

Medium Field Strength (0.35 T)
1, right ventricle
2, left ventricle
3, mitral valve
4, left atrium
5, atrial septal defect
6, right atrium
7, right coronary artery

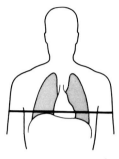

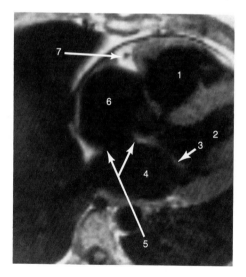

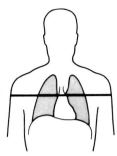

Medium Field Strength (0.35 T)
1, ascending aorta
2, main pulmonary artery
3, patent ductus arteriosus
4, descending aorta
5, superior vena cava

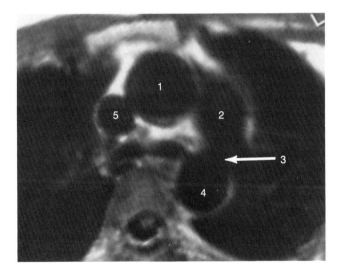

Medium Field Strength (0.35 T)
1, ascending aorta
2, main pulmonary artery
3, mass
4, descending left pulmonary artery
5, descending aorta
6, right pulmonary artery
7, superior vena cava

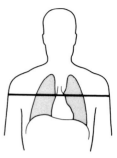

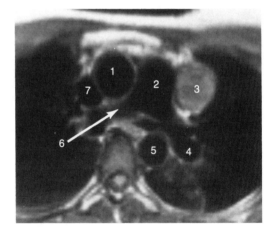

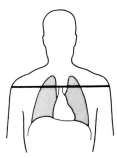

Medium Field Strength (0.35 T)
1, dilated ascending aorta
2, absent main pulmonary artery
3, hypoplastic left pulmonary artery
4, left main bronchus
5, right-sided descending aorta
6, right main bronchus
7, hypoplastic right pulmonary artery
8, superior vena cava

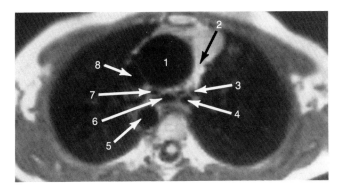

Medium Field Strength (0.35 T)
1, hypertrophied right ventricular wall
2, left ventricle
3, descending aorta
4, inferior vena cava entering right atrium
5, right atrium
6, pericardium

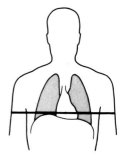

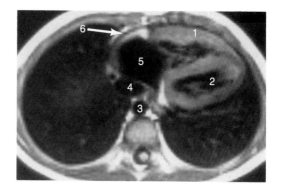

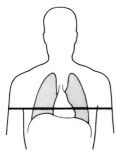

Medium Field Strength (0.35 T)
1, hypertrophied right ventricular wall
2, ventricular septal defect
3, left ventricle
4, right-sided descending aorta
5, left atrium
6, right atrium

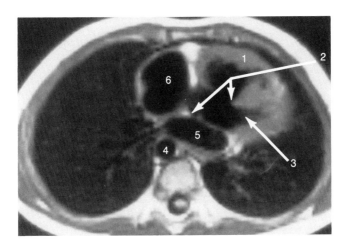

Medium Field Strength (0.35 T)

1, ascending aorta at level of sinuses of Valsalva
2, right ventricular outflow region
3, left atrium
4, superior vena cava
5, pericardial hematoma

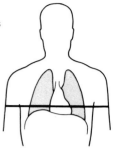

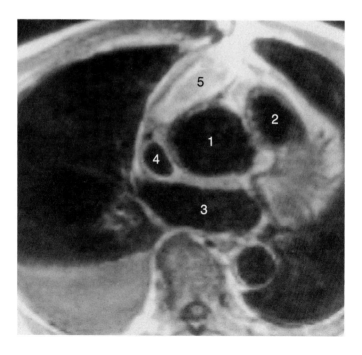

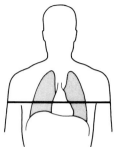

Medium Field Strength (0.35 T)
1, right ventricle
2, ventricular septum convex toward
   left ventricle
3, left ventricle
4, descending aorta
5, pleural effusion
6, right atrium
7, pericardial thickening

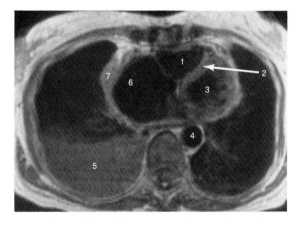

Pericardial thickening in the presence of a "box shaped" heart with small ventricles and large atria suggests constrictive pericarditis. Bowing of ventricular septum toward left ventricle, right atrial enlargement, and right pleural effusion are due to elevated right heart pressures.

Medium Field Strength (0.35 T)

1, right ventricle
2, bright signal in false aortic lumen due to slow flow and entry-slice phenomenon[a]
3, true aortic lumen
4, left atrium
5, level of aortic valve
6, right atrial appendage

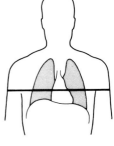

[a]See: Bradley, W.G., Jr. (1988): Flow phenomena in MR imaging. *AJR*, 150:983–994.

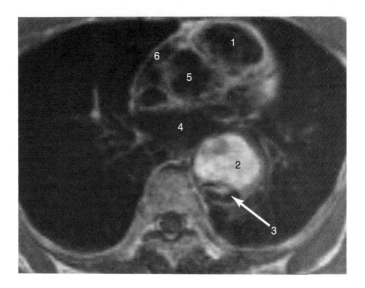

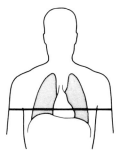

Medium Field Strength (0.35 T)
1, right ventricle
2, left ventricle
3, false aortic lumen
4, intimal flap
5, true aortic lumen
6, left atrium
7, right atrium

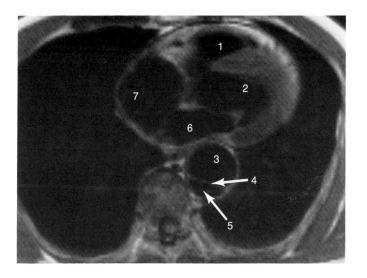

**Hypertrophic Cardiomyopathy
with Ventricular Septum
Thickened Out of Proportion to
Lateral Wall of Left Ventricle/
Medium Field Strength (0.35 T)**

1, focally thickened ventricular
    septum
2, left ventricle
3, right atrium
4, right ventricle

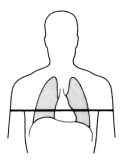

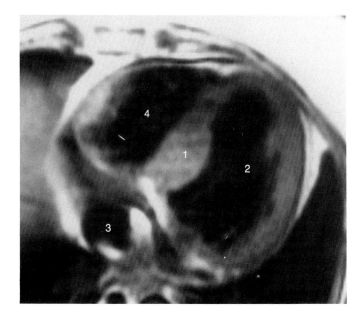

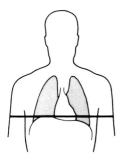

Malignant Giant Cell Tumor of Bone Metastatic to Left Atrium/ Medium Field Strength (0.35 T)
1, ascending aorta
2, right ventricular outflow region
3, metastasis to left atrium

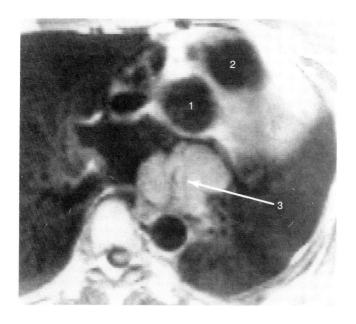